I0101418

All About
ALZHEIMER'S DISEASE

By Laura Flynn R.N., B.N., M.B.A., in consultation with her nurse educator associates and physicians who assisted in contributing and editing.

ISBN No: 978 1 896616 55 1

© 2011, 2017 Mediscript Communications Inc.

The publisher, Mediscript Communications Inc., acknowledges the financial support of the Government of Canada through the Canadian Book Fund for our publishing activities.

Printed in Canada

Book and Front Cover design by:
Brian Adamson, www.AdamsonGraphics.net

AL1002010

ALL ABOUT BOOKS
Trusted • Reliable • Certified

- 40+ titles available
- Comply with accreditation and regulatory bodies
- Suitable for caregivers, boomers with elderly parents, health workers, auxiliary health staff & patients
- Self study style with "test yourself" section
- Health On the Net (HON) certified

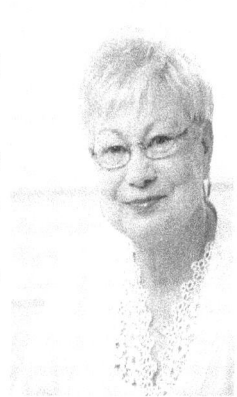

Some of our titles:

Alzheimers Disease	Arthritis	Multiple Sclerosis
Pain	Strokes	Elder Abuse
Falls Prevention	Incontinence	Nutrition & Aging
Personal Care	Positioning	Confusion
Transferring people	Care of the Back	Skin Care

For complete list of titles go to www.mediscript.net

Contact: 1 800 773 5088
Fax 1800 639 3186 • Email; mediscript30@yahoo.ca

CONTENTS

INTRODUCTION

This book provides basic, non controversial and trusted information that can help a wide spectrum of readers.

The primary objective of the information is to help a person provide effective quality care to a loved one or someone in his or her care.

Your role as a caregiver could mean the older person in your care is a family member or loved one, or you may be a non family member who is helping out a friend. Alternatively, you may be a paid health worker providing quality care for a client. With this in mind, we will alternate between referring to family members, loved ones, older persons and clients.

All the information is reliable and was written by a group of eminent nurse educators who ensured the information complies with best practice guidelines and satisfies the various accreditation and regulatory bodies. Because there is so much unreliable information on the internet, you can be assured the "All About" publications are HON (Health On the Net) certified.

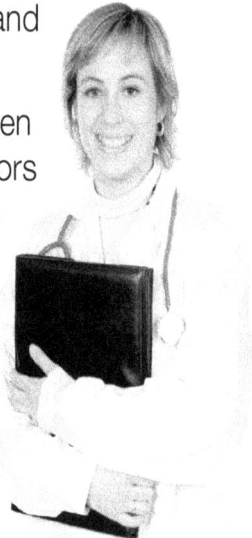

This book can be an invaluable aid to:

- A caregiver caring for a relative or friend;
- A health worker seeking a reference aid;
- Any person involved in health care wishing to expand his or her knowledge

---

SOMETHING TO THINK ABOUT...

When I was young, I admired clever people.
Now that I am old, I admire kind people.

Abraham Heschel

AN IMPORTANT MESSAGE
FROM THE PUBLISHER

Each person's treatment, advice, medical aids, physical therapy and other approaches to health care are unique and highly dependant upon the diagnosis and overall assessment by the medical team.

We emphasize therefore that the information within this book is not a substitute for the advice and treatment from a health care professional.

This book provides generic information concerning Alzheimer's disease, the causes and symptoms, and common sense well established care practices for caring for people with the condition.

With all this in mind, the publishers and authors disclaim any responsibility for any adverse effects resulting directly or indirectly from the suggestions contained within this book or from any misunderstanding of the content on the part of the reader.

HAVE YOU HEARD

Two healthcare workers and their supervisor from a small nursing home were taking a lunch break in the break room. In walked a beautiful woman dressed in silk scarves and wearing large polished stone jewelry.

"I am 'Gina the Great'," she said. "I am so pleased with the way you have taken care of my aunt that I will now grant the next three wishes!"

With a wave of her hand and a puff of smoke, the room filled with flowers, fruit, and bottles of drink, proving that she did have the power to grant wishes before any of the nurses could think otherwise.

The first healthcare worker spoke up. "I wish I were on a tropical island beach," she said. With a puff of smoke, she was gone.

The second healthcare worker spoke next: "I wish I were rich and retired and spending my days traveling to ski resorts." With a puff of smoke, she, too, was gone.

"Now, what is the last wish?" Gina the Great asked the supervisor.

The supervisor looked around the room and then she said, "I want those two back on the unit by the end of the lunch break."

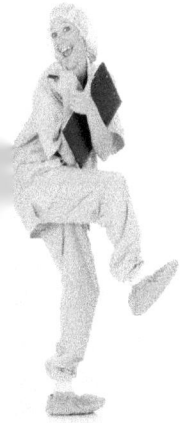

HOW MUCH DO YOU KNOW

It helps to figure out how much you know before you start. In this way you will have an idea as to the gaps in your knowledge prior to reading the content. Please circle to indicate the best answer. Remember, at this stage, you are not expected to know all the answers:

1. Which statement about AD is correct?

a. It is a temporary condition.

b. There is no genetic relationship to AD.

c. AD rarely affects communication.

d. The only certain way to diagnose it is by autopsy.

2. Which of the following is a controllable risk factor for AD?

a. Age

b. Sex

c. Family history

d. Serious head injury

3. Which symptom is included in the ten warning signs for AD?

a. Difficulty with eating

b. Wandering behaviour

c. Problems with abstract thinking

d. Inability to speak except for a few simple words

4. Which strategy would be most helpful for you to use at mealtime for a person with AD?

a. Use nonbreakable dishes

b. Play loud music during mealtime

c. Ensure the person eats three big meals each day

d. Put all the food servings on the table at one time

5. Which statement about AD is true?

a. It occurs only in older people

b. Medication can cure the disease

c. It occurs only in persons with a genetic defect

d. It is the most common form of dementia

6. What percentage of persons with AD in the U.S. are cared for at home?

a. 10%

b. 40%

c. 70%

d. 90%

7. Which technique would help to improve communication with the person who has AD?

a. Speak in a loud voice

b. Give him plenty of choices

c. Approach him from the side

d. Maintain eye contact while talking to him

ANSWERS

1. d. The only way to be absolutely certain of Alzheimer's is by way of an autopsy.

2. d. A head injury is the only controllable risk factor.

3. c. Abstract thinking becomes difficult, especially when it comes to remembering.

4. a. This takes away potential problems of safety and waste.

5. d. The majority of dementia symptoms can be linked to AD.

6. c. 70% and growing.

7. d. Maintain eye contact. The other three suggestions are not recommended.

WHAT IS ALZHEIMER'S DISEASE? (AD)

This book provides an overview of Alzheimer's disease (AD) and can help to increase your understanding of how to provide quality care to a family member with the condition. If you work with older people, it is likely that you have already cared for someone with AD. If not, you may soon be assigned to care for a person with this disease as it is becoming very common in our society.

AD occurs most often in older persons. As the percentage of older persons in society increases, more and more people are getting the disease. Some famous people who have been diagnosed with AD are Ronald Reagan (former President of the United States), Rita Hayworth (actress), and Sugar Ray Robinson (middleweight world champion boxer). It has been estimated that over 4.5 million Americans have AD. There are currently about half a million Canadians living with Alzheimer's disease or a related dementia. Estimates for Canada are that one in 11 persons in the 65+ age category has the disease. As well, the incidence in persons 85 years and more is 25%.

Alzheimer's disease is not a new disorder. In 1906, a physician, Dr. Alois Alzheimer, found changes in the brain of a 51-year-old woman who had died of a strange mental illness. The condition was found to be a new disease and was later named "Alzheimer's disease" after its discoverer.

Dementia describes a group of symptoms caused by a variety of disorders. The disorders cause a decline in mental and cognitive function over time. AD is the most common form of dementia, resulting in the death of certain types of nerve cells in the brain. It affects thought, memory, and language. Changes occur in the way a person behaves, as well as in mood and personality. Judgment and reasoning are affected as well as the ability to communicate and to carry out daily activities.

When a person presents with symptoms of AD, tests are usually done to detect other possible causes of dementia. Once other problems have been ruled out, diagnosis depends heavily upon the person's history. The only certain way to diagnose the disease requires an examination of the brain tissue at autopsy. Research is ongoing into the cause and treatment of AD. There is no cure for the disease, although medication can prevent or reduce some of the symptoms, at least for some time. These medications work best when used along with behavior management. The basis of care for people with AD remains behavior management.

WHAT CAUSES ALZHEIMER`S DISEASE?

The exact cause of AD is not known. Researchers are exploring possible causes, contributing factors and treatments for the disease. A number of risk factors seem to make it more likely that someone will get the disease. Some of these factors are:

- Age. This is the greatest known risk factor for AD. The disease is uncommon before the age of 65. After the age of 65, however, the incidence doubles every 5 years.

- Family history and genetics. Having someone in the immediate family (i.e. parent or sibling) with AD increases a person's chances of getting the disease.

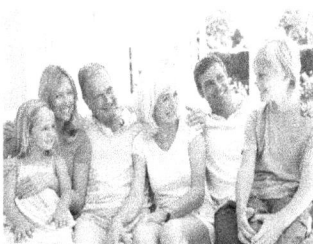

The more individuals with AD in a family, the higher the risk for remaining family members. Certain types of genes cause forms of AD that may occur even before the age of 65. A rare form of inherited AD can occur as early as the age of 30.

The risk factors of age, family history and genetics cannot be controlled. Scientists are also exploring risk factors that can possibly be controlled to prevent AD. These include:

- Environment. Studies indicate that AD may develop partly as a result of environmental influences. For example, having a twin with AD puts the other twin at increased risk but it does not mean that the disease will definitely occur.

- Serious head injury. There seems to be a link between serious head injury and later onset of AD.

- Lifestyle choices, such as a balanced diet, active social life, avoidance of tobacco and alcohol, and regular physical and mental exercise, promote a healthy brain and may protect against AD.

- Factors related to blood circulation, such as high blood pressure or high cholesterol, heart disease, stroke, and diabetes appear to increase the risk of AD.

AD is more common in women but that may be because women tend to live longer than men in our society. It is likely that the disease is caused by a number of factors that are present at the same time, rather than just one.

SYMPTOMS OF ALZHEIMER'S DISEASE

Memory changes with aging happen to everyone. People with AD, however, have severe problems with reasoning, memory and language. These changes seriously affect the person's ability to work, to communicate with others and to care for himself. The Alzheimer's Association has developed a list of ten warning signs that help to show the difference between changes due to aging and those due to AD. These warning signs are:

1. Memory loss. The person with AD forgets recently obtained information.

2. Difficulty performing familiar tasks. Even simple everyday tasks are hard for the person with AD to complete.

3. Problems with language. The person with AD often has trouble finding the correct word for even common items such as a toothbrush.

4. Disorientation to time and place (e.g. forgetting what day it is, getting lost) happens often.

5. Poor or decreased judgment. The person with AD may show poor judgment in many aspects of everyday life (e.g. dresses oddly, gives away valuable belongings).

6. Problems with abstract thinking. Handling personal finances (e.g. not paying the bills, paying too much for purchases) becomes a struggle.

7. Misplaced belongings. Items may be often lost or placed in odd places.

8. Changes in mood or behavior. Rapid mood swings (e.g. crying, aggression) with no obvious reason may be common.

9. Changes in personality. Confusion, suspicion, withdrawal may be evident.

10. Loss of initiative. Some people with AD may sleep for long periods of time and not want to do much of anything when awake.

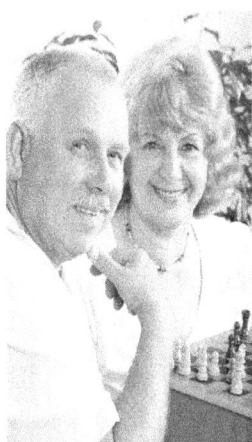

AD starts out slowly and worsens over time. Different methods of staging have been used to show how the disease progresses. One staging system divides the disease process into seven stages. Another system uses three stages – early, middle, and late – to describe the common changes that occur as the disease progresses over time. Keep in mind that the symptoms occur at different times for persons with AD. As well, symptoms from one stage often overlap with symptoms from another stage of the disease. The three-stage system is described below:

Early stage

Symptoms in the early stage coincide with the warning signs outlined by the Alzheimer's Association. Mild forgetfulness is one of the first signs of AD. Although this happens to all of us at some time, it happens more often to someone with AD. The person may forget names, appointments, and telephone numbers.

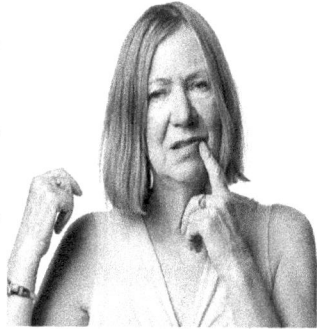

Someone with AD will have difficulty with new learning and the memory problems will worsen over time. The person may forget the correct names of simple everyday objects. Items may be forgotten or misplaced. For example, the newspaper may be placed in the refrigerator or the butter in the laundry basket. At first, the person with AD will be concerned about the memory lapses and decreasing ability to perform tasks that were once easily completed. This knowledge may cause a great deal of stress.

Judgment may be impaired. The ability to do well in demanding job situations will decrease. Help may be needed with handling money and performing tasks that require abstract thinking. Some of the other symptoms common at this stage include trouble concentrating, getting lost easily, and forgetting the date and time. Shifts in mood, restlessness, anxiety, and mild coordination problems may also occur.

CONSIDER FOR A MOMENT...

Forgetfulness is an early sign of AD. The person with AD may even forget how to get to a location that was once very familiar, or may be able to get there and then forget how to find the way back. Have you ever been in a situation where you could not find your way? If so, how long did the experience last? How did you feel about it? How do you think the person with AD might feel in a similar situation?

Middle stage

At this stage, the person with AD will have great trouble organizing her thoughts. The person forgets where she is and doesn't remember what day or month it is. Sleep may be disturbed and the person may mix up day and night. Wandering behavior is common. Sexual behavior may be inappropriate. Memory worsens to the point that the AD individual may no longer know her family members. Help with simple tasks like dressing, bathing, and toileting will be needed.

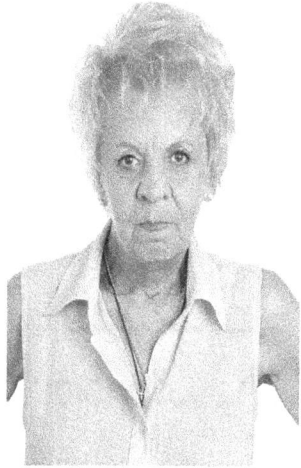

Marked personality changes become apparent over time. Rapid changes in mood, such as aggression or severe anxiety, can happen for no obvious reason. The person may be suspicious and experience delusions. The personality changes and challenging behaviors may cause a great deal of anxiety for family members and healthcare workers.

Late stage

As the disease advances, the person with AD may become unable to walk or to speak, except for possibly a few simple words. There may be difficulties with eating. The ability to remember will be lost and the person will require help with all aspects of personal care. Loss of bowel and bladder control occurs.

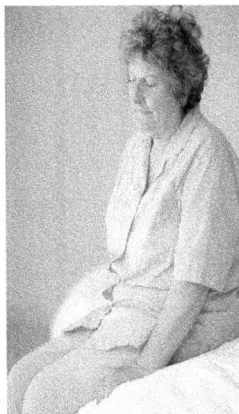

Even though physical and mental abilities have decreased greatly at this stage, there may be a reaction to music and touch. There may also be some response to emotion.

People with AD generally live for eight to 12 years following diagnosis. However, this time frame can vary greatly with some people living 20 years or more with the disease.

CONSIDER FOR A MOMENT ...
Have you ever cared for
someone with AD?
If so, what symptoms
have you observed?

CARING FOR SOMEONE
WITH ALZHEIMER'S DISEASE

In most cases, a person is diagnosed with AD while living at home and remains there during the earliest stages of the disease. Family members are often heavily involved in the care of their relative at this point. A home health aide may visit and assist with care and the family may use respite services as available. Other health providers besides the physician may be involved in caregiving. These include the nurse, social worker, physical therapist, occupational therapist, nutritionist, clergy, and others as appropriate to the person's situation.

As the disease progresses, challenging behaviors associated with AD become more pronounced and the family may no longer be able to provide the care that is needed. At this point, the family may explore placement into a care facility. Possible options include assisted living facilities, personal care homes, centers that specialize in the care of clients with dementia, and nursing homes.

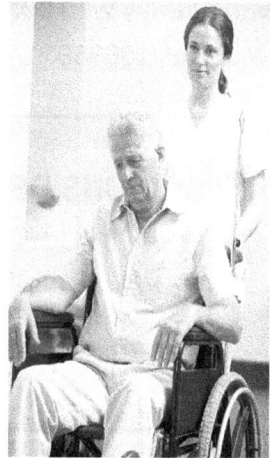

General care

The type of support and care you give to a person with AD depends on how far the disease has advanced and also on her individual needs. Over time, she will require greater assistance with all aspects of daily living. Check the care plan to find out more about the care of your loved one. Consult with your health care professional if you have concerns about your family member's behavior or if you do not understand any aspect of the care plan. This section discusses general approaches to care that have been found to be helpful in the care of people with AD.

The person with AD will display many challenging behaviors such as wandering, agitation, and aggression. When your loved one displays challenging behaviors, consider the situation. Examine his behavior. What is happening? Try to see the behavior from his point of view. For example, repeatedly calling a relative on the phone may seem logical to the person who cannot remember any of the calls he recently made. Consider if the behavior is harmful to anyone; if not, it may be okay to ignore it.

Consider what factors (e.g. fatigue, noise) may have led up to the behavior. Is this person scared, hungry, tired, or uncomfortable? Is the environment noisy and crowded? Where possible, take steps to remove the source of anxiety. Sometimes resolving the problem is as easy as taking the person to the bathroom. At other times, you may have to try different approaches to find one that works.

Despite the progressive loss of memory, judgment, and other abilities, many persons with AD retain some interest and ability in old hobbies and skills for a period of time. The math teacher who cannot remember his own name may be able to recall the numbers to open the doors to a locked unit. The woman who loved the piano may be able to play simple tunes despite obvious progression of the disease in other areas. The devoutly religious person may be able to take part in church services or may find it comforting just to watch.

Several basic factors to keep in mind when caring for someone with AD are:

- Always treat the person with respect and dignity. Treat people with AD the same way that you would like to be treated or as you would like someone to treat one of your loved ones.

- Be flexible in the care that you give. Things will often go more smoothly if you adjust your schedule to meet the needs of the person with AD.

- Do not argue, correct or confront the person. Instead, try to redirect problem behaviors into more positive forms. People with AD are generally easily distracted. For instance, if your loved one is creating a lot of noise by banging a spoon on the table at mealtime, you may be able to get him to pay attention to something else. Several possible options are:

- Remind him to use the spoon to eat the dessert.

- Replace the spoon with another item.

- Take him for a short walk.

- Keep things simple. Break complex tasks into simple steps. For example, if you want the person to sit at the kitchen table to eat, tell her to "Sit on the chair," "Pick up the spoon," and so on.

- Establish routines. Where possible, have these routines similar to what the person finds familiar.

- Establish reminders. It may be useful to put a picture of a toilet on the door to the bathroom as a reminder.

- Limit choices to two possible answers (e.g. the red dress or the blue one). Both answers should be acceptable.

- Encourage independence as long as possible. Encourage hair combing, washing, and going to the bathroom. Over time, the amount of help the person needs to do these simple tasks will increase and the time will come when she will be unable to do them at all.

- Promote hobbies and skills of interest.

- Ensure that your loved one gets adequate rest each day.

Don't force care on people who are resistive. Remember, your health care professional and the care plan are valuable resources. If you are not familiar with the person, check with others who are. Medications can be used to control some of the challenging behaviors common with AD. They will work better, however, when used with other strategies such as a flexible approach.

Communications

Some challenging behaviors may occur because of poor communications between you and the person with AD. Here are some tips that you may find helpful:

- Ensure that the surroundings are quiet.

- Approach the person from the front so that you will be easily seen and he or she will not be startled.

- Stay at eye level with the person. Sit down if he is seated and stand up if he is standing.

- Before you begin speaking, look directly at the person and smile. People with AD are often able to detect tension and stress in others. Make sure that the nonverbal cues (smiles, body language) that you send are reassuring. Use a calm and friendly tone of voice.

- Speak in a normal tone of voice.

- Slow down. Speak clearly and slowly so as not to confuse the person with AD. It may be necessary to repeat what you have said.

- Use words that are simple and familiar in everyday language.

- Use your hands to point or demonstrate as you are talking.

- Ask closed-ended rather than open-ended questions. Closed-ended questions can be answered simply (e.g. "yes" or "no"). An example of a closed-ended question is "Do you want a drink of water now?" Open-ended questions such as "How are you?" can be very confusing and even frustrating for people with AD. As the disease progresses, AD sufferers are unable to organize their thoughts to be able to answer open-ended questions.

- Give your family member lots of time to answer any questions.

- Avoid the word "don't." Whenever possible, state things in a positive way. For instance, if the person is not chewing his food well at mealtime, you could remind him to eat slowly, rather than saying, "Don't eat so fast." Follow up with smiles and encouragement when he does so.

- Repeat important information as needed.

- Touch can be very calming when you are talking to the person with AD. Place your hand on her arm or your arm around her shoulders as you communicate in a calm and unhurried manner.

Mealtime

Several challenges can occur with respect to eating for people with AD. They may forget to eat or be unable to let you know when they are hungry or thirsty. Frequent small meals or snacks may work better than three big meals a day. Encourage them to eat and drink throughout the day.

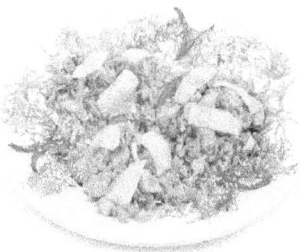

People with AD will forget how to eat in a socially acceptable way at mealtime. They may not be able to understand the purpose of food or how to use knives, forks, and spoons. A noisy room may make them too anxious to eat. Finger foods such as fruit, sandwiches, or vegetables allow the person to stay independent with feeding as long as possible. Provide a mug or cup with a wide handle that she can use for drinking. Serve one food at a time. Give simple directions and praise:

"Open your mouth."

"Good."

"Now swallow."

"You're doing very well."

Check the person's teeth and mouth when you provide morning care each day. The person with AD will not always be able to tell you when decayed teeth or inflamed gums are causing a problem. Ensure he has dentures in and is wearing glasses if used.

Below are suggestions to follow to prevent injuries from occurring at mealtime:

- Ensure that the table is not cluttered.
- Use nonbreakable dishes if necessary.
- Remove harmful items from the table.
- Ensure sure that food is cut into small pieces (to prevent choking).
- Check the temperature of the food before you serve it.

Report any concerns you may have about swallowing or possible choking.

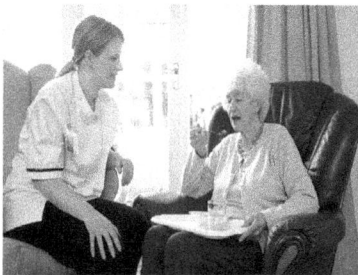

Bathing

As AD advances, your family member will need help with all aspects of personal hygiene. She will need your help to wash her hands, to bathe, to brush her teeth, to toilet and so on. Without good personal hygiene, people are at risk for skin breakdown and infection. Bathing people with AD often poses particular challenges for caregivers. Try to make bath time a relaxing experience. Play soft music, ensure the room is warm, and make sure that you have plenty of time so that you are not rushed. Being organized in your work will help the procedure to go more smoothly. Check that:

- You have closed the door to ensure privacy.

- You have another person available to assist as needed.

- The temperature of the water and room is comfortable.

- You have everything you need, such as soap, washcloth, and towel, laid out ahead of time.

Other tips that may help with bathing include:

- Give one direction at a time.

- Allow the person to get into the bath slowly.

- Explain what you are going to do before you do it.

- Give the person a washcloth to hold onto during the bath.

- Allow him to wash himself without help as much as possible.

- Use a calm and encouraging approach. Smile and praise the person.

- Demonstrate what you wish him to do; for example, wash his face.

Many people with AD dislike bathing. They may be afraid of water or may not understand what is happening. Perhaps the person is not feeling well or the room is chilly. Some people will strongly resist bathing. They may strike out, scream and try in every way to stop the process. Don't force the person to get in the tub or shower. Be flexible. Remember that each situation and person is unique. Give some thought to what is happening and why. Consider the options that are available to you. For example, is your family member refusing to undress due to modesty? If so, can you bathe him with underwear on or with a towel wrapped around him? People with AD are often fearful of getting water around their face and head. Can you schedule bathing and hair washing at different times? Consider bathing the person later in the day or giving a sponge bath.

A towel bath has been found to be helpful for some confused people who resist personal care. The process involves placing washcloths and towels in a plastic bag and then adding warm water with no-rinse body shampoo to the bag. Using the towels and washcloths, the healthcare worker begins the cleansing procedure at the person's feet moving upwards. The upper body and the hands are washed last.

This bathing process provides warmth, comfort, and relaxation while cleansing in a manner that is not too invasive. If your loved one will tolerate the presence of two caregivers, one of you can talk to her and help distract her while the other performs the bathing.

One aspect of personal hygiene that is often overlooked for people with AD is mouth care. Good mouth care can prevent cavities and gum disease. People with AD should see a dentist on a regular basis and their teeth need to be brushed twice a day. If dentures are used, ensure they are cleaned each night. A variety of products and strategies are available for mouth care for confused and debilitated people. A dentist or dental hygienist may need to be consulted.

CONSIDER FOR A MOMENT ...

Can you think of any other strategies that may help make bathing a more enjoyable experience for the person with AD? Have you tried strategies in the past other than those mentioned above? If so, which ones worked well? Why do you think that was?

Toileting

As the disease progresses, AD will affect bladder and bowel control. As with most other aspects of care for the person with AD, it is important to be flexible with toileting. The following tips may help you to care for his or her toileting needs:

- Ensure that the bathroom is easy to find. Keep the path to the bathroom well lit. It may be necessary to post a sign to help the person remember where the bathroom is located.

- Remind him regularly to go to the bathroom.

- Monitor the toileting pattern and develop a schedule.

- Watch for cues (e.g. grimacing or agitation) that he needs to go to the bathroom.

- Make sure that clothing is easy to remove.

- If the person needs help with starting to void (urinate), try running the water for a while.

- Observe how well he gets on and off the toilet. Is it necessary to have handrails put on? Be patient when accidents occur. If accidents do continue, protective pads, liners or briefs may be needed.

- Assist with hand washing following toileting.

Safety

You can help make the environment safer for an AD sufferer. Some general suggestions are outlined below.

- Use grab-bars for the bathtub.
- Keep medications out of reach.
- Use a non-slip mat for the bathtub.
- Ensure that proper lighting is in place.
- To prevent falls, ensure that the person wears proper footwear.
- Remove items such as sharp objects that can injure the person.
- Check scatter rugs and remove if necessary to prevent tripping.
- Supervise when the person is smoking or lock away the cigarettes and lighter.
- Remove cleaning solutions and personal care items (e.g. soap, shampoo) that could be harmful if ingested. Many people do not realize that common household plants can also be poisonous.

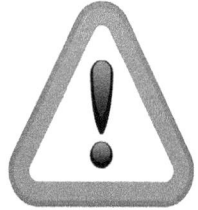

If your loved one is living at home, it may be necessary to lock away guns, power tools, and electrical appliances. Alcohol must be kept out of reach and unused outlets covered with safety plugs.

Wandering

Another important safety issue for people with AD is wandering. Confused people who wander away from home or a care facility are at extreme risk of injury. If you are caring for a wandering person at home, supervise her closely and keep exterior doors locked. Alarms may have to be installed. You may decide to use a bracelet with your loved one's name, address, and telephone number on it. Check with your local chapter/office of the national Alzheimer's Association (US) or the Alzheimer Society of Canada to find out about available resources, including a registry/ enrolment program for wandering persons.

Most facilities caring for people with AD have secured units for residents who wander. The units are locked and an alarm sounds when at risk clients leave the unit. Follow agency policies with respect to supervision and locking of doors.

As a caregiver, you are in an excellent position to identify potential safety issues before they become major problems. If you think that the safety of your family member may be at risk, and you are not sure what to do about it, get advice from a health care professional.

CASE EXAMPLE

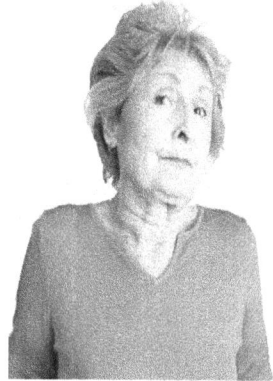

Barbara, 69, lives with her husband of forty years. They have one son, John, who lives nearby. Barbara has been active in church and community work over the past twenty years. The Browns have many friends in the neighborhood and have led a very active social life.

Some time ago, her husband noticed that his wife often forgot things, such as where she placed her eyeglasses or her sweater. Once, a neighbor invited them to dinner. Barbara graciously accepted the invitation, but then promptly forgot all about it. On another occasion, she got the invitation date wrong and the couple arrived at a party at a friend's house a day early.

John first became puzzled when he noticed that his mother repeatedly left items at his home when she came to visit. He spoke to his father about it who explained that John's mother was busy with community work and tended to be a little forgetful at times. Still, John felt uneasy.

One day, John dropped in to his parent's home for

an unexpected visit. He had not seen his mother for some time and he found her behavior to be quite odd. Barbara wanted to make coffee but could not remember where she had put the coffee pot. She could not recall the names of some common household items and seemed to have trouble following the conversation.

As time went on, even John's father had to admit that something was wrong. Barbara left a pot cooking on the stove when she went out one day. She insisted on shopping for groceries but regularly came back with just a couple of items. Always careful with her appearance, her attire became scruffy and odd. Once "the life of the party", she now avoided social events. She finally consented to see her family doctor. To everyone's dismay, she was ultimately diagnosed with AD.

Which of the ten warning signs of AD has Mrs. Brown displayed?

How do you think Mrs. Brown's physician was able to make a diagnosis of AD?

YOUR ANSWERS TO CASE EXAMPLE

SUGGESTED ANSWERS TO CASE EXAMPLE

Which of the ten warning signs of AD has Barbara displayed?

The warning signs of AD that Barbara displayed include:

- Decreased judgment (unusual dress)
- Misplaced belongings (e.g. sweater, eyeglasses)
- Problems with language (finding the correct words)
- Difficulty performing familiar tasks (e.g. grocery shopping)
- Possible change in personality (withdrawing from social functions)
- Memory loss (forgetting recently attained information such as dates of social functions)

How do you think Barbara's physician was able to make a diagnosis of AD?

Barbara's physician probably did tests to detect other possible causes of dementia. Once other problems were ruled out, diagnosis was made based on Barbara's history. The only certain way to diagnose the disease requires an examination of the brain tissue at autopsy.

CONCLUSION

AD is a form of dementia that is becoming much more common as the population ages. The exact cause of the condition is unknown although a variety of factors make it more likely that someone will contract the disease. AD progresses slowly and has been described through a three-stage process. Research is ongoing into the cause and treatment of AD. There is no cure for the disease, although medication is available to prevent or reduce some of the symptoms, at least for a while. Various approaches and strategies have been found helpful in the care of people with AD but behavior management remains the basis of care.

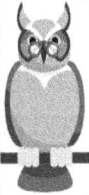

CHECK YOUR KNOWLEDGE

1. Name two risk factors for AD

2. Identify three common symptoms in the early stages of AD

3. Identify three basic factors to keep in mind when caring for someone with AD

4. Give three strategies that you could use to communicate with someone with AD

5. Identify two strategies you could use to make bath time more pleasant

6. Identify three strategies you could use to make the environment safer for someone with AD

TEST YOURSELF

Please circle to indicate the best answer:

1. What statement would be most appropriate to make to a person with AD who is eating food from another person's tray at mealtime?

a. Don't do that

b. Stop that right now

c. That is very poor behaviour

d. Here, eat the vegetables on your plate

2. Which symptoms best describe a person in the late stage of AD?

a. Wandering

b. Misplacing belongings

c. Trouble finding the correct word for items

d. Confined to bed, not able to speak (except possibly a few words)

3. You are caring for someone with AD who is resisting getting into the tub. He has an unpleasant body odor and has not had a tub bath in over a week. Which of the following strategies would be most appropriate for you to follow?

a. Try a sponge bath

b. Leave him alone and try again next week

c. Find another person to help you force him into the tub

d. Try to convince him that a tub bath would be beneficial at this time

4. Which of the following is a common symptom of AD?

a. Pain

b. Headaches

c. Changes in mood

d. High blood pressure

5. Which strategy would be most helpful in caring for an agitated person who has AD?

a. Try to determine the cause of the agitation

b. Explain that the behavior is upsetting to others and must stop

c. Encourage the person to find out more about stress management techniques

d. Have a lengthy discussion with the person to try and find the source of the problem

6. Which item poses a possible safety hazard to the person with AD who is cared for at home?

a. Plants in the kitchen

b. Grab bar in the bathroom

c. Non-slip mat for the bathtub

d. Cigarettes out of the person's reach

7. You are caring for someone in the middle stage of AD. Which strategy would NOT be helpful with respect to toileting of this person?

a. Ensure the bathroom is easy to find

b. Make sure that clothing is easy to remove

c. Watch for cues that the person needs to go to the bathroom

d. Wait until the person tells you she needs to use the bathroom

ANSWERS

1. d. Do not argue, correct or confront the person. Instead, try and redirect problem behaviors into more positive forms. People with AD are generally easily distracted.

2. d. As the disease advances, the person with AD may become unable to walk or to speak, and will probably be confined to bed.

3. a. Consider bathing the person later in the day or giving a sponge bath.

4. c. Rapid mood swings (e.g. crying, aggression) with no obvious reason may be common.

5. a. Consider what factors may have led up to the behavior. Where possible, take steps to remove the source of anxiety.

6. a. Many people do not realize that common household plants can be poisonous.

7. d. As the disease progresses, AD will affect bladder and bowel control. You should remind the person regularly to go to the bathroom.

REFERENCES

Alzheimer Society of Canada (2006a). Alzheimer disease and risk factors. Retrieved May 29, 2006, http://www.alzheimer.ca/english/disease/causes-riskfac.htm

Alzheimer Society of Canada (2006b). The three stages. Retrieved May 29, 2006, http://www.alzheimer.ca/english/disease/progression-3stages.htm

Alzheimer Society of Canada (2006c). The progression of Alzheimer's disease. Retrieved May 29, 2006, http://www.alzheimer.ca/english/disease/progression-intro.htm

Alzheimer Society of Canada (2006d). Daily living. Retrieved May 29, 2006, http://www.alzheimer.ca/english/care/intro.htm

Alzheimer's Association (2006a). Causes. Retrieved May 17, 2006, http://www.alz.org/AboutAD/causes.asp

Alzheimer's Association (2006b). 10 warning signs of Alzheimer's disease. Retrieved May 17, 2006, http://www.alz.org/AboutAD/causes.asp

Alzheimer's Association (2006c). Statistics about Alzheimer's disease. Retrieved May 17, 2006, http://www.alz.org/AboutAD/Statistics.asp

Alzheimer's Disease Education and Referral Center [ADEAR]. (2006a). General information. Retrieved May 17, 2006, http://www.nia.nih.gov/Alzheimers/AlzheimersInformation/GeneralInfo/#howmany

Alzheimer's Disease Education and Referral Center [ADEAR]. (2006b). Caregiver's guide. Retrieved May 17, 2006, http://www.nia.nih.gov/Alzheimers/Publications/caregiverguide.htm#wandering

Ebersole P., Hess P., Touhy T. and Jett K. (2005). Gerontological nursing healthy aging. 2nd Ed. St. Louis: Elsevior Mosby.

Mayhew, M. (2005a). The growing challenge of Alzheimer's disease: Part 1. The Journal for Nurse Practitioners, 1 (2), 74-83.

Nash, J. (2000, July 17). The new science of Alzheimer's. Time, 32-39.

Schindel Martin, S., Morden, P. and McDowell, C. (1999). Using the towel bath to give tender care in dementia: A case example. Perspectives, 23(1), 8-11.

Sorrentino, S. (2004). Mosby's Canadian textbook for the support worker. Toronto, ON: Mosby.

www.ingramcontent.com/pod-product-compliance
Lightning Source LLC
Chambersburg PA
CBHW071343290326
41933CB00040B/2196